The Physical Th.

TREATING
ANKLE SPRAINS
AND STRAINS

*Complete with Prevention
and Rehabilitation Strategies*

Ben Shatto, PT, DPT, OCS, CSCS

Publishing services provided by

Archangel Ink

ISBN-10: 1548116890

ISBN-13: 978-1548116897

CONTENTS

AUTHOR'S NOTE

This rehabilitation guide has been written and categorized into very specific sections that target different aspects and time periods during a person's injury and recovery process. Although it's best to read this rehabilitation guide in sequential order, it can also be used as a reference guide for specific aspects of ankle sprains and strains injury or recovery. For example, you may initially only be interested in reading the **Return to Full Activity and Sport** section while someone else may only be interested in reading the **Acute Phase of Rehabilitation**.

There are certain aspects of each section that may have repeated information because the rehabilitation guide is written in such a way that information can be independently read. I intentionally created the content this way in order to make it easier for those that will choose to read the sections out of sequence on an as needed basis.

The treatment advice and information is based upon my clinical experience and the present research. As information and best practice patterns evolve, the advice in this guidebook may evolve as well.

Throughout this rehabilitation guide, I reference books, products, supplements, topical agents, and web sites that I personally use and recommend to my family, friends, clients, and patients (for use in the clinical setting). For your reference and convenience, please refer to the **Resource Guide**.

INTRODUCTION

Ankle sprains and strains are a common everyday occurrence. In most cases, the injuries are nothing more than a nuisance that temporarily affects your training and mobility. However, severe cases can lead to lengthy rehabilitation and even surgery.

Knowing how to effectively self-treat and manage ankle sprains and strains is important in order to resume your training and normal activities without the risk of additional damage, injury or re-injury. *When you can confidently self-treat, you can limit pain levels, return to activity faster, and prevent reoccurrences.*

Proper muscle strength and proprioception of the lower leg and foot is important to limit future injury. As you stretch, stress, and strengthen around the new scar tissue, you may find that it's not strong enough to cope with your increasing physical demand. *This is why a properly coached and graded rehabilitation plan is critical.* A proper rehabilitation from the initial injury to the full return to sport and/or activity must include a full return to strength, mobility, and balance.

So then, what is the best course of action to take upon spraining your ankle? Beginning with the acute phase of rehabilitation, I will walk you through the treatment plan on how to rehabilitate your ankle through the intermediate (sub-acute) phase of rehabilitation and return to full activity and sport.

ANKLE SPRAINS AND STRAINS

If you walk, jog, run or generally spend time on your feet, you're likely to experience an ankle sprain at some point. Ankle sprains are the most common orthopaedic injury. They are a common occurrence and can happen to anyone at any age. Most of the time, ankle sprains will not require specific medical treatment. However, knowledge of the best methods to self-manage this injury is extremely helpful. When you can confidently self-treat, you can limit pain levels, return to activity faster, save money on costly physician and rehabilitation bills and prevent reoccurrences.

The *Journal of Sports Medicine* (January 2014) conducted a meta-analysis on the topic of ankle sprains. The findings concluded that women were at higher risk of ankle sprains and that children were more likely to sprain an ankle than an adolescent or an adult. Indoor and court sports were the highest risk activity. However, an ankle sprain can occur just as easy from stepping off a curb, sliding off your bed or accidentally stepping on a pet or child's toy.

Often in the case of an ankle injury, there is both a sprain and a strain. A sprain is an injury to the ligament. Ligaments connect bones to other bones. Strains are injuries to muscles or tendons. In most cases of an ankle injury, you can assume that there was an injury to both a ligament and muscle. The course of treatment is nearly identical whether there was or wasn't a sprain and/or a strain.

In general, an ankle sprain occurs when you twist your ankle too far. It causes the ligaments (which support the ankle) to get stretched and/or torn. Depending on the severity and the ligament damaged, a sprain may take from several weeks to months to fully heal. The more pain and swelling and bruising you experience initially often indicates the severity of the injury, possibly indicating a longer recovery.

A chronically sprained or severely sprained ankle that isn't properly treated could present with ligament deficiencies. This means that one or more of the ligaments in the ankle were completely torn or significantly over stretched. In cases such as these, the individual can learn to compensate by utilizing muscle strength and motor control in order to manage pain and discomfort while maintaining mobility. In some cases, surgical intervention will be required to repair the torn ligaments.

Proper treatment is the key to insure that you completely recover from the injury. Otherwise, you're at risk for repeated injury when you don't complete the necessary course of rehabilitation. Once you have experienced an ankle sprain, you are more likely to experience another one if you don't properly rehabilitate your ankle and address any precipitating factors that may increase your risk of repeated injury.

Many different types of ankle sprains are possible, but the most common sprain is known as the **lateral ankle sprain**. Initially during a lateral ankle sprain, the foot rolls inward (inverts) farther than it should which causes a "sprain" of the lateral ligaments of the ankle. It may also affect the lateral muscles or tendons of the ankle which produce eversion of the foot causing a strain. The muscles most typically affected are known as the peroneals. In more severe cases, the fibula bone or the fifth metatarsal bone near the pinky toe could also be injured either with a fracture or the tendon could rupture from the bone.

Ankle Sprains

Inversion **Normal** **Eversion**

Sprained Lateral Ligament

Sprained Medial Ligament

A **medial sprain** occurs when the foot rolls too far outward or into eversion. This type of injury affects the inside portion of the ankle. This injury is common in contact sports. It can happen when one person's foot is planted and contact from another player pushes the leg inward which causes a relative outward motion onto the ankle.

Typically, the fibula tends to block this motion. Therefore, if a sprain occurs, an accompanying fibular fracture is often also present.

Another type of sprain that can occur is known as a **syndesmosis sprain** or the high ankle sprain. The syndesmosis is the fascia and ligamentous tissue that holds the tibia and fibular together. This type of sprain accounts for about 15% of all ankle sprain injuries. This type of injury is most common in collision sports such as American football. Typically the foot is rotated externally (outward) and loaded right when a collision occurs which results in an injury of the tissue that connects the two bones. Another mechanism of injury occurs when the foot is overly flexed up which causes the two bones to splay too far apart.

Many of the treatment modalities outlined in this rehabilitation guide will be geared toward addressing **lateral ankle sprains**. However, most of the treatment advice can be applied to any type of ankle sprain or strain. In many cases, a similar treatment approach can be utilized for a fibular fracture, for a fibular fracture with surgical fixation injuries or other foot/ankle injuries. (One must take into account any potential weight bearing issues or wound care that may need to be performed in cases of surgical intervention.) Any special consideration for a particular type of injury and treatment advice, such as in the case of a syndesmosis sprain and a particular method of taping for a high ankle sprain, will be dually noted.

GRADING ANKLE SPRAINS AND STRAINS

Sprains

Sprains are categorized as Grade I, II, or III. A **Grade I sprain** is the most common. It's typically associated with only mild damage to the ligament, and instability doesn't affect the joint. There is typically mild tenderness over the injury site and swelling.

A **Grade II sprain** is a partial tear to the ligament and is usually associated with some laxity (hypermobility). Bruising on or near the site of injury may appear. There will be significant tenderness over the injury site and moderate pain and swelling. If this occurs, it's best to wear a brace for several weeks. Ideally, scar tissue will form and compensate for the lax (over stretched) ligament, so the joint doesn't become hypermobile.

Proper muscle strength and proprioception of the lower foot is important to limit future sprains. Proprioception is a term used to describe the body's ability to use tiny receptors in the muscles, tissues, and joints of the body to determine where it is in space. For example, through proprioception when you close your eyes you still know what your arm is doing.

A properly trained physician, physical therapist or athletic trainer can usually determine the likely grade of sprain present and the ligaments involved. An X-ray may be indicated to rule out other concomitant injury such as an associated fibular or fifth metatarsal fracture.

In **Grade III sprains,** a full tear of the ligament occurred. There is typically severe swelling and bruising along with notable ankle instability. One typically consults with an orthopaedic surgeon for possible repair. After surgery, a guided physical therapy program is recommended.

Lateral ankle sprain

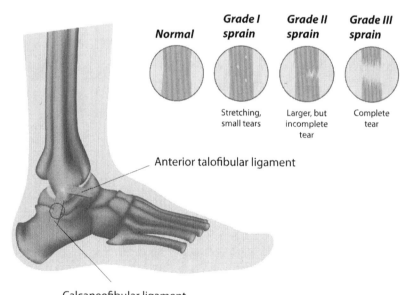

Strains

Like sprains, strains are also categorized as Grade I, II, or III.

A minor strain is classified as a **Grade I tear**, whereas a complete rupture, or tear, is classified as a **Grade III tear**. **Grade II tears** are partial ruptures or tears. Severe Grade II and Grade III tears cause impaired muscle function and usually have associated bruising that occurs near the site of injury. Grade I injuries tend to be mild in that they tend to heal fully. With proper care and rehabilitation, the healing times can be reduced. Grade II tears can often be rehabilitated as well although the healing time is longer. Grade III tears may require surgical intervention.

PHASES OF HEALING

I t's important to understand how your body heals and what processes take place during the different phases of healing. The different phases of healing include: **bleeding, inflammation, proliferation, maturation**, and **remodeling**.

Understanding what is happening in the body's tissues during these phases is critical in guiding treatment throughout any rehabilitation process. The different phases or stages are not mutually exclusive and overlap considerably. Depending on treatment methods and activities, you can influence the outcomes either positively or negatively.

The following descriptions of the different phases of healing and rehabilitation will help you understand not only which processes are occurring, but also how to best self-treat.

Acute – Protection Phase

The acute stage of rehabilitation, also initially known as the protection phase for the first several days post injury, is correlated with the **bleeding and inflammation phase** of healing. The healing process begins right away by bleeding. In order to prevent any further damage, the body's response is to limit all movement by swelling and spasming (splinting) muscles.

During the bleeding and initial inflammatory phase, many important inflammatory chemicals are released into the bloodstream to the area of injury. This initial inflammatory response is a critical component to healing the damaged area. Inflammation is only problematic if it becomes chronic or too severe which can cause further tissue damage.

A soft tissue injury is termed as acute from the initial time of injury and during the worst of the pain, bleeding, and swelling. The usual time frame for acute initial symptoms to occur is two to four days post injury. This can vary depending on how you treat your injury. The acute phase of rehabilitation often takes much longer.

The focus of treatment at this stage is to **protect** your injury from further damage from movement and activity or other treatment modalities. Avoid excessive activity and tissue mobilization.

A common mistake is to take medications that can negatively impact the healing. This doesn't allow the body the opportunity to fully complete this stage. I recommend that you don't start taking an anti-inflammatory medication unless your swelling is out of control. Although the swelling should be limited, don't eliminate it completely as your body needs to process through each phase of healing.

Sub-Acute – Repair Phase

The sub-acute phase of rehabilitation typically correlates with the **proliferation phase**. During this phase, the body is progressing with the healing of the injury. A soft tissue injury is termed as sub-acute when the initial acute phase transitions into the repair of the injured tissues. This phase of tissue healing as well as rehabilitation starts three to six days post injury when your body starts to make new or heal the injured tissues. This phase commonly lasts up to six weeks.

During this phase, your body is eliminating waste materials that may be present from the initial injury. It's also starting the healing process by bringing in nutrients and a mixture of extracellular matrix and collagen to make new tissue. The development of a new network of blood vessels, if needed, will replace the damaged ones (a process called angiogenesis).

From a rehabilitation standpoint, this is the most critical phase in order to insure a speedy recovery. The aim is to reduce the need to protect your injury as the new scar tissue begins to mature and strengthen. It's also an important time to provide your body with all of the necessary resources to heal quickly and completely. The rehabilitation goal is to help your body produce the strongest scar tissue possible while limiting loss of function when taking steps to prevent future re-injury.

Late Stage – Remodeling Phase

The late stage or remodeling phase is often correlated with the end of the sub-acute phase of rehabilitation and the return to sport phase of rehabilitation. During the **remodeling phase**, your body continues to heal and remodel the damaged tissue. Healing is a continuum. This phase starts between six and eight weeks post injury and will last three months or more.

At this stage, your healing tissue is reasonably mature but as you stretch, stress, and strengthen around the new scar tissue you may find that it's not strong enough to cope with your increasing physical demand. This is why a properly coached and graded rehabilitation plan is critical. Although it may appear that the injury has finished healing when maturation phase begins, it's important to keep up with the treatment plan.

If the injury site and the treatment plan are neglected, there is risk of the injury site breaking down because it's not at its optimal strength (which could cause re-injury). Even after maturation, injury sites remain up to twenty percent weaker than they were initially. A proper rehabilitation from the initial injury to the full return to sport and/or activity must include a full return to strength, mobility, and balance.

Your body can detect if a repaired structure is still weaker than necessary. It will either learn to compensate, which can lead to re-injury or cause excessive stress elsewhere that increases the risk of injury, or it will stimulate additional new tissue to help strengthen and support the healing tissue. Proper rehabilitation and training allows you to meet the demands of normal exercise and functions safely *without* the risk of re-injury.

Chronic Phase – Ongoing Repair and Remodeling

Beyond three months is referred to as the chronic phase. In cases of severe injury, it's not uncommon for this phase to be combined with the **remodeling phase** for up to six to twelve months post-injury. This phase correlates to the return to sport and activity phase of the rehabilitation process.

Soft tissue is constantly being affected with micro-trauma from your daily activities and workouts. This stimulates the body to repair and remodel the tissue to meet your specific exercise demands. This is the whole reason why people train. This is in essence the **Overload Principle**, and why it's a critical component to training. The body needs to sustain a sufficient stimulus to "overload" the tissues and stimulate the tissue to grow stronger. In the case of injury, the "overload" went too far. The goal of training is "overload" the tissue with just the right amount of stimulus to produce the desired training effect.

ACUTE PHASE OF REHABILITATION

At the time of injury, you may often feel or hear a popping sound. This is followed by a fairly rapid onset of swelling in the ankle, typically along the lateral (outside) part of the ankle near the bump known as the lateral malleolus. The swelling can be present throughout the entire ankle and even part way up your leg. This is also usually associated with a significant amount of pain.

Depending on the severity of the pain, the location of the swelling, and any potential bruising, your course of treatment may vary. *If you are unsure as to the severity of the sprain, suspect other severe injury (such as a fracture), and/or are experiencing severe pain, please seek competent advice from a medical doctor, physical therapist or athletic trainer.*

Depending on how the injury occurred and the severity of pain, an X-ray may be appropriate to determine if there was any potential bone fracture. If a fracture occurred, the initial acute phase of treatment would be different (likely a period of time being immobilized) and the entire acute phase prolonged. The recovery afterward may also vary slightly, but it could generally follow the course of treatment outlined below.

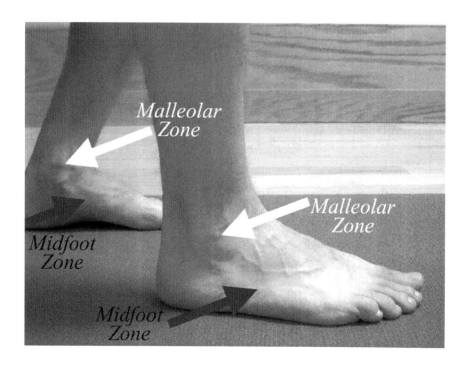

The **Ottawa Ankle and Foot Rules** offer guidance on when and if an ankle or foot injury should have an X-ray. An X-ray is indicated only if a person has pain in the *Malleolar Zone (see white arrows)* and any of the following findings: bone tenderness at lateral or medial malleolus or the inability to bear weight (four steps) immediately after injury. A foot X-ray is indicated only if a patient has pain in the *Midfoot Zone (see black arrows)* and any of the following findings: bone tenderness at the base of the fifth metatarsal or navicular bone or the inability to bear weight (four steps) immediately after injury.

The focus of treatment during the acute phase is to **protect** your injury from further damage from movement and activity or other treatment modalities. Initially, you may wear an air splint, ACE wrap or some other lace-up or slip-on style brace to help with stability, inflammation, and pain control of the ankle. In severe cases, a walking boot or cast may be necessary if there is a severe Grade II or III injury. You may even need to use an assistive device, such as crutches, to limit the amount of pressure placed on the ankle.

In most cases of a typical **lateral ankle sprain**, you will transition from wearing the brace as soon as the initial pain subsides. The goal is to return to full motion as soon as possible once the risk of further damage has been eliminated.

If you have a **Grade II sprain**, you may choose to wear a splint for several weeks. Your ankle and the specific ligament injured will hopefully stiffen and this will help prevent the ligament from not becoming overly lax and/or stretched which reduces the risk of re-injury.

In the case of a **syndesmosis sprain** (or the high ankle sprain), limit any weight bearing activities during the initial phase of recovery. You may also potentially need to limit weight bearing during the sub-acute phase of rehabilitation. You can also use tape or a strap to help reduce the stress on the injured tissues.

Initial Treatment

The initial course of treatment following the sprain includes **PRICE**, which stands for **P**rotection, **R**est, **I**ce, **C**ompression, and **E**levation.

- **PROTECT** – Initially, you may choose to "protect" the injury site. This may include the use of a splint, walking boot or cast, and/or crutches. Even using a simple ACE wrap is a method of protecting the site from further injury. Refrain from an activity that may have caused the injury. Try not to over rotate or move the injured area.

- **REST** – In this case, rest would indicate not using the ankle. I would initially recommend using a crutch or crutches to either fully unweight the ankle (or at least take some pressure off) when walking (particularly in the case of a syndesmosis sprain). Remember, your body must rest in order to heal. Having adequate rest is critical for recovery.

- **ICE** – Apply ice to the ankle, and the sooner, the better. *The rule for icing is to apply ice no more than twenty minutes per hour.* Do not place the ice directly against the skin, especially if you are using a gel pack style. Individuals with poor circulation or impaired sensation should take particular care when icing. A bag of frozen peas can be ideal. If you have one, utilize a cold therapy machine that circulates cool water over the injury site.

- **COMPRESSION** – Compression helps to prevent and decrease swelling. Swelling can cause increased pain and slow the healing response if it becomes too severe. Limit it as much as possible. You can utilize a common ACE wrap or you can purchase a pair of mild over-the-counter compression socks. If you have a friend who is medically trained, many different taping techniques can also assist in decreasing swelling and bruising if present. Many physical therapists or athletic trainers can apply Kinesiology Tape for you or you can find application techniques online. In **Ankle Self-Taping Strategies**, I demonstrate a specific technique to help with swelling. There are many other possible techniques to assist with pain control or stability. I have had luck using **KT TAPE**, **RockTape**, **Kinesiology Tape**, and **Mummy Tape** brands.

- **ELEVATION** – Elevate means to keep the ankle above the level of the heart. This allows for gravity to assist in keeping the inflammation and swelling down. Typically, I would combine the ice with compression and elevation.

The initial goal of treatment during the **Protection Phase** is to reduce pain, limit swelling, and avoid re-injury or further damage. During the **Protection Phase**, your chance of a full recovery will be increased if you avoid the following factors referred to as **HARMS** during the first 48 to 72 hours post-injury.

- **HEAT** increases swelling and bleeding. Avoid heat packs, a hot bath, and saunas.

- **ALCOHOL** increases swelling and bleeding by thinning the blood. Too much alcohol can delay the healing response.

- **RUNNING**, exercise, or any activity that aggravates the injury can increase pain, swelling, and bleeding. Always check with a health professional prior to resuming your sport or activity.

- **MASSAGE** and tissue mobilization can increase swelling and bleeding. Direct mobilization to the injured area may aggravate the damaged tissues. Avoid mobilization for the first 48 to 72 hours (unless you are specifically trained in how to perform the right type of mobilization). During the initial injury, a lymphatic massage or an indirect massage (away from the injury site) may be helpful. Please consult your health practitioner for the best advice for your injury.

- **SMOKING** has been proven to reduce the healing response. If you avoid smoking throughout your recovery, the healing time will be reduced.

After the 48 to 72 hours post-injury, you will progress out of the **Protection Phase**. The following Acute Phase should last no more than seven to ten days (with the exception of severe injuries).

The **Acute Phase** can overlap with the **Sub-Acute Phase** of healing as well. Understanding the **Phases of Healing** is important because it guides treatment throughout the rehabilitation process.

However, there will be a variation on how fast you progress from one rehabilitation phase to another. Variation in healing times is based on many treatment variables including: the severity of the injury; your age; prior health and/or activity status; current activity status; nutritional factors; and how your body heals.

Gentle Movement

Gentle movement can help to reduce swelling. The motion helps your body bring in much needed nutrients into the site of injury which aids in healing. During the acute phase and after the initial protection phase, move your ankle as much as you can tolerate, but don't be aggressive with the movement. Don't move your ankle if it causes more than a mild to moderate increase in pain. This may irritate the injury and cause further swelling and inflammation. Movement is good and helpful unless it causes severe pain.

Focus on the up and down movement of your ankle (known as plantarflexion and dorsiflexion). Avoid the side to side motion (known as inversion and eversion). The goal is to gain your full range of motion (ROM) back as soon as possible without causing more damage. Avoid any extreme movements, particularly side to side, so that you don't stress or stretch an already over-stretched ligament. Keep within a normal amount of motion and avoid extreme end ranges.

Range of Motion (ROM)

Start to increase the range of motion (ROM) of your ankle. Initially, work to progress the plantarflexion and dorsiflexion movement (the forward and backward movement of the ankle). (As your pain subsides, you can progress to side to side motion as well as all other motions.)

Always start with the easier exercise before progressing to the more difficult exercise. Exercises should always be relatively pain free with no more than a minor increase in discomfort.

Start with a very easy exercise, **Ankle Pumps**. Just pump your ankle forward and backward into plantarflexion and dorsiflexion movement. Perform 10-15 repetitions several times a day on both feet.

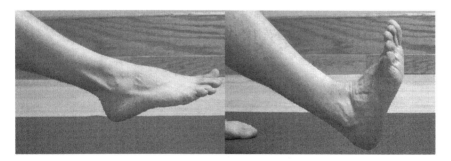

A slightly more aggressive method to regain dorsiflexion and to stretch the Achilles tendon is to use a strap. Be sure that you don't experience more than a mild increase in pain with any of the advised movements or stretches.

For the **Foot and Ankle Stretch with a Strap**, place a strap (or belt) around the bottom of your foot. Pull your toes, foot, and ankle upward toward your shin until you feel a stretch in the bottom of your foot and/or your calf muscles. This stretch is best performed barefoot, but it can be performed with shoes on. Perform 1-2 minutes on each leg, 2 or 3 times per day.

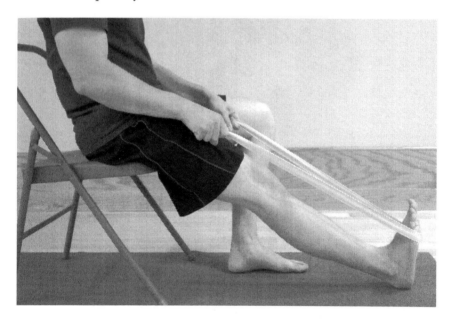

Supplementation

During the acute phase, I recommend starting at least a thirty day course of **CapraFlex** by Mt. Capra. CapraFlex is an organic glucosamine and chondroitin supplement which also includes an herbal

and spice formulation designed to naturally decrease inflammation and support healing. Since it takes a little longer to build up in your system, it shouldn't disrupt the initial critical inflammatory healing factors.

I recommend CapraFlex to anyone recovering from an injury or attempting to prevent injury when performing at a very high level. I personally use it, and in my practice, it has helped clients recover faster and prevent injury.

CapraFlex can interfere with some blood thinning medication, so if you are on this type of medication, please check with your physician. Also, if you're allergic to goat based products, this one is not for you as it contains goat protein. (I prefer goat based protein products because the size of the protein is the most similar to our own.)

Like CapraFlex, **Tissue Rejuvenator by Hammer Nutrition** contains glucosamine and chondroitin as well as a host of herbs, spices, and enzymes to help support tissues and limit inflammation. I recommend taking either CapraFlex **OR** Tissue Rejuvenator.

I also recommend a colostrum supplement called **CapraColostrum** by Mt. Capra *(also a goat based product)*. Colostrum is the first milk produced by female mammals after giving birth. It contains a host of immunoglobulins, anti-microbial peptides, and other growth factors. It's especially good at strengthening the intestinal lining which prevents and heals conditions associated with a leaky gut. Colostrum can also help a person more effectively exercise in hotter conditions. Over all, it can boost the immune system, assist with intestinal issues, and help the body to recover faster.

You can take CapraColostrum independently or in conjunction with either CapraFlex **OR** Tissue Rejuvenator. I recommend taking these supplements as a recovery strategy. I recommend initially trying a 30 day protocol. If the supplements are aiding your recovery, you may choose to continue taking them for an additional 30 days. I implement this protocol as part of a prevention strategy during times of heavy volume or high intensity training.

Healthy Eating

Your body tissue needs nutrients to be able to perform at a high level. *Eat for performance.* Your food is your fuel, and the old adage is true. You are what you eat. Avoid processed food as much as possible. *Whenever possible, eat nutrient rich foods.* No empty calories. Limit sugary food and add more healthy protein and healthy fat in your diet. Maintaining a diet with adequate healthy fats is essential in providing the nutrients to support all hormone function in the body as well as support the brain and nervous system. Adequate protein intake is necessary to support muscle health and development.

Pain Relief

- In some cases, the use of an electronic device such as a TENS machine may also assist your early pain relief. TENS is an abbreviation of **TRANSCUTANEOUS ELECTRICAL NERVE STIMULATION**. A TENS units works on the theory that your skin and sensory receptors conduct sensation faster than pain fibers, so by utilizing an electrical device, such as a TENS unit, the perception of pain can be reduced.

TENS machines can be an excellent short term adjunct to help control pain. Please consult with your physician or healthcare practitioner.

- **TOPICAL ANALGESICS.** There are many topical agents which can be used for pain. My two favorites to help manage pain and stiffness are **Arnica Rub** (an herbal rub) and **Biofreeze**. Use liberally. These help with pain, but they don't get to the source of the pain. In addition, consider icing as it can help to reduce pain levels as well.

- **ORAL MAGNESIUM.** Although you can increase the magnesium in your diet by eating foods higher in magnesium such as spinach, artichokes, and dates, I recommend that you take **Mag Glycinate** in pill form. Taking additional magnesium (particularly at night) can help to reduce pain. It is also very helpful in reducing overall muscle soreness and aiding in a better night's rest. I recommend beginning with a dose of 200 mg (before bedtime) and increasing the dose as needed. I would caution you that taking too much magnesium can lead to diarrhea. Mag Glycinate in its oral form is the most highly absorbable. Although not as absorbable, **Thorne Research Magnesium Citrate** and magnesium oxide can also be beneficial.

Magnesium is known to help decrease pain and soreness. Try a magnesium ice soak. Add the magnesium flakes to either cold or ice water. Although the magnesium flakes will not absorb as well in the water, you still get the benefit of the magnesium and cryotherapy (the use of extreme cold as medical therapy). Options include: **Epsoak Epson Salt** or **Ancient Minerals**

Magnesium Bath Flakes. I find that the magnesium flakes work better, but they are significantly more expensive than Epson salt.

- **ACUPUNCTURE.** I am personally a big fan of acupuncture. It's very useful in treating all kinds of medical conditions. Acupuncture has been shown to be very effective for pain relief. It can be particularly effective in treating pain as it addresses the issues on multiple layers. Acupuncture treatment may even help with the initial swelling as acupuncture affects the nervous system response which may affect blood flow patterns and may even stimulate the healing response.

- **ASK FOR HELP.** If you are unsure as to the severity of the sprain, suspect other severe injury (such as a fracture), and/or are experiencing severe pain, please seek competent advice from a healthcare practitioner. Seek a qualified and competent physician, physical therapist, athletic trainer or sports chiropractor who specializes in working with athletic clients.

  The **American Physical Therapy Association** offers a wonderful resource to help find a physical therapist in your area. In most states, you can seek physical therapy advice without a medical doctor's referral (although it may be a good idea to seek your physician's opinion as well).

Rehabilitation Recap for the Acute Ankle Sprain

The initial course of treatment includes **PRICE** (**P**rotect, **R**est, **I**ce, **C**ompression, and **E**levation).

Slowly attempt to regain limited mobility and range of motion (ROM) in your ankle. Be sure to **rest** and take **pain relieving measures**.

Your body needs quality **healthy food and nutrients** to help it heal. Consider **supplementation** in order to insure that your body has the necessary nutrients for a speedy recovery.

Be as active as you can, but don't over stress the injury. If the injury is more severe, you may need to limit mobility and weight bearing temporarily.

Prior to progressing to the sub-acute phase of rehabilitation, insure the following:

- You should be able to stand with equal weight on both feet and not experience a significant increase in pain.
- The swelling in and around the ankle and lower leg is manageable.
- You can walk (although the ankle is likely stiff).
- You don't have any other injury that would require medical management.

The initial acute phase of an ankle sprain can last one to seven days on average. Severe cases may take longer. If you are unsure on how to progress your rehabilitation, be sure to ask for help.

INTERMEDIATE (SUB-ACUTE) PHASE OF REHABILITATION

As you enter into the intermediate phase of rehabilitation or the sub-acute phase of the injury, it has likely been three to ten days since your initial injury. This phase of rehabilitation can last from seven days to many weeks before progressing into the final phase of rehabilitation (and ultimately, back to full function).

The intermediate or sub-acute phase of rehabilitation will correlate with different phases of healing including the **repair phase** and the **proliferation phase** which can last up to about six weeks. Near the end of the intermediate/sub-acute rehabilitation phase, you may even be in the **remodeling phase** or **maturation phase** of healing. This starts between six and eight weeks post injury and will last three months or more as your body continues to heal and remodel the damaged tissue. Healing is a continuum. The phases of healing may overlap. They tend to correlate with phases of rehabilitation, but each phase will not conform exactly to the other.

Are You Ready?

Prior to initiating the rehabilitation protocol for the intermediate (sub-acute) phase, you should be able to:

- Stand with equal weight on your feet and not experience an increase in ankle pain.

- Walk (although the ankle is likely stiff).

This phase will include activity and active treatments. Each individual's recovery is different. The amount of time you spend on each exercise or activity will vary.

During this phase, you will:

- Progress your walking back to normal.

- Progress your range of motion (ROM).

- Start gentle resistive exercises.

- Initiate proprioceptive and balance exercises. (Proprioception is a fancy word that describes your nervous system recognizing where your body is in space. This is how you know what your extremities are doing even if your eyes are closed.)

During this phase, continue with the strategies outlined in the **Acute Phase of Rehabilitation** which includes: swelling management (PRICE); rest; supplementation; and pain relief. Progressing from the out of the intermediate (sub-acute) phase of rehabilitation is always symptom dependent.

Walking

At this time, the focus will be to normalize your walking pattern. This means that you have a proper heel strike, which includes rolling onto the foot into full weight bearing on the leg, and then propelling forward with a toe off. The focus is to normalize your gait pattern without significantly increasing your pain level or causing excessive swelling.

If you have been walking, then increase the amount of weight you have been putting on the ankle and foot.

If you have been using a crutch to unweight the foot, then start the progression of increasing weight bearing during walking. You will continue to use the crutch as long as needed until you can walk nearly normal without limping. The goal is normal ambulation until you can walk without a limp. It's better to utilize the crutch to unweight the leg and foot only as much as necessary to perform a nearly normal walk or gait sequence.

Range of Motion (ROM)

Start to increase the range of motion (ROM) of your ankle. Initially, work to progress the plantarflexion and dorsiflexion movement (the forward and backward movement of the ankle). (As your pain subsides, you can progress to side to side motion as well as all other motions.) It is important to get full dorsiflexion ROM back as soon as possible. So in almost all cases there should be extra focus on regaining dorsiflexion first.

Always start with the easier exercise before progressing to the more difficult exercise. Exercises should always be relatively pain free with no more than a minor increase in discomfort.

RECOMMENDED EXERCISES:

Start with a very easy exercise, **Ankle Pumps**. Just pump your ankle forward and backward into plantarflexion and dorsiflexion movement. Perform 10-15 repetitions several times a day on both feet.

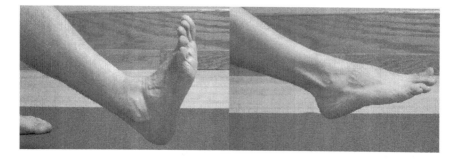

Ankle Alphabet is another recommended exercise. Move your foot and ankle only by pretending that your big toe is a pen. Draw the alphabet using capital letters. Perform 1-2 times a day.

Be somewhat gentle while stretching your calf *(as demonstrated below)*. These stretches shouldn't cause more than a mild increase in pain or discomfort. Start with the strap, and progress into standing as pain allows.

Foot and Ankle Stretch with a Strap

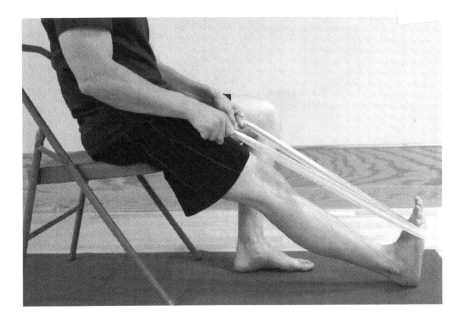

» Place a strap (or belt) around the bottom of your foot. Pull your toes, foot, and ankle upward toward your shin until you feel a stretch in the bottom of your foot and/or your calf muscles. This stretch is best performed barefoot, but it can be performed with shoes on.

» Perform 1-2 minutes on each leg, 2 or 3 times per day.

Calf Stretch - Gastrocnemius

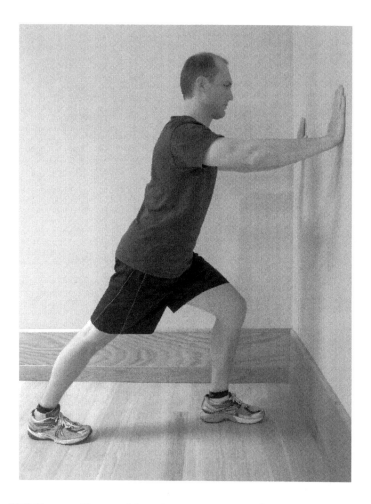

» While standing and leaning against a wall or counter, place one foot back behind you and bend the front knee until a gentle stretch is felt on the back of the lower leg. Maintain a good upright posture.

» Your back knee should be straight the entire time, with your heel on the ground.

» Hold for 30 seconds, and 3 repetitions per side.

Calf Stretch - Soleus

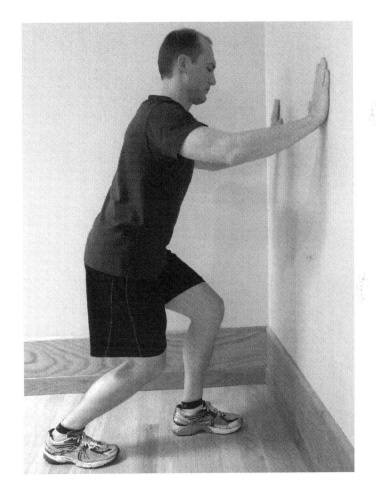

» While standing and leaning against a wall or counter, place one foot back behind you and bend the front knee until a gentle stretch is felt on the back of the lower leg. Maintain a good upright posture.

» Your back knee should be bent the entire time, with your heel on the ground.

» Hold for 30 seconds, and 3 repetitions per side.

Self-Subtalar Mobilization

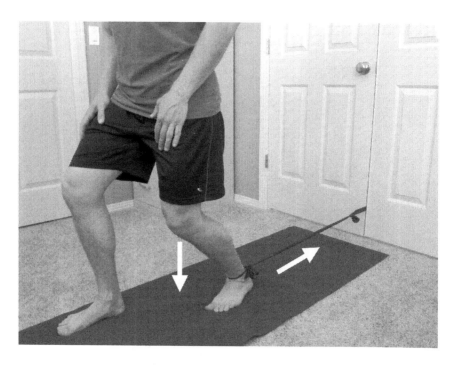

» Attach a thicker exercise or mobility band to a solid surface. Place the band lower on the involved ankle with the affected side back behind you. Bend your front knee until you feel a gentle stretch on the back of your lower leg. Maintain a good upright posture.

» Your back knee should be bent the entire time with your heel on the ground. Gently oscillate while you feel a stretch in the calf and the band pulls your ankle posteriorly.

» Hold for 30 seconds, and complete 3 repetitions.

Mobility/Compression Bands for Ankle Sprains

Mobility bands, such as **Rogue Fitness VooDoo X Bands** and **EDGE Mobility Bands**, are gaining in popularity as a self-treatment tool. The use of mobility bands affects blood flow to the area and speeds up healing. Mobility bands also help reset some of the receptor cells in the muscle tissue that cause excessive muscle tightness. There are different methods and theories as to how to utilize the mobility band. The specific technique varies according to the injury.

In the case of an ankle sprain, the mobility band can improve range of motion (ROM) and help to decrease swelling and pain. The key is to wrap the mobility band more lightly than in other treatment techniques in order to avoid restricting blood flow. The mobility band would be wrapped with approximately 25% stretch or less.

The entire treatment should last only a couple of minutes. If you start to experience numbness, tingling, excessive pain or your foot turns completely white, please discontinue the treatment. Remove the mobility band, and move your ankle back and forth while performing ankle dorsiflexion and plantarflexion.

This technique can be used in the case of a high ankle sprain. If you are utilizing the circumferential taping technique, be sure that the tape is intact prior to performing this technique. Please refer to **Ankle Self-Taping Strategies – Circumferential Taping for High Ankle Sprains**.

(If you suffer from any form of blood clotting disorder or are on blood thinning medications, I would advise against utilizing mobility bands for any type of aggressive, deep compression.)

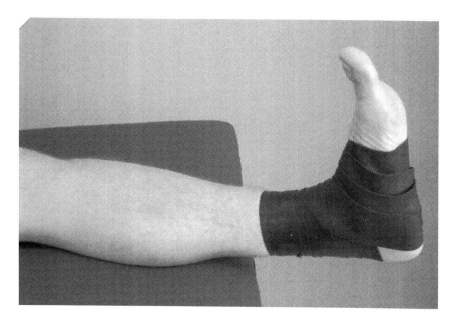

» Starting **mid foot,** wrap the mobility band with 25% stretch. Tuck the end of the mobility band inside the part that has already wrapped.

» Sit with your ankle unsupported and free floating.

Mid Foot Variation – Part 2

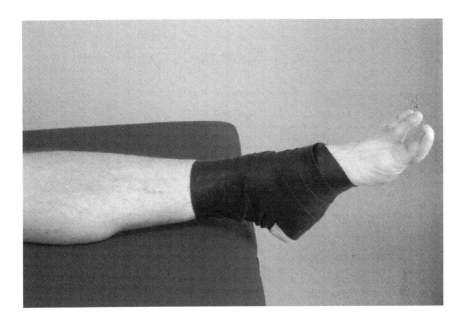

» With the mobility band in place, pump your ankle back and forth for as much motion as possible in each direction.

» Perform for approximately 30-60 seconds or for approximately 15-30 repetitions.

Ankle Self-Taping Strategies – Posterior Fibular Glide

Posterior Fibular Glide – Part 1

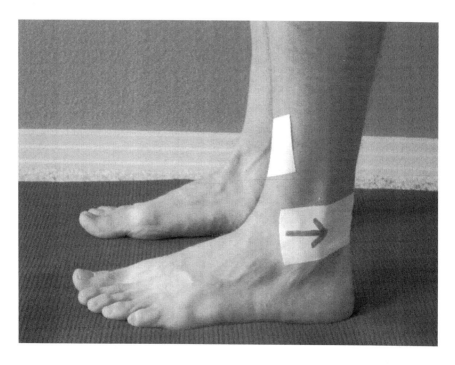

» Position the athletic tape slightly in front of the lateral malleolus of the injured ankle. The malleolus is the large bump on the side of the ankle which is actually part of the fibular bone.

» Take the tape about half of an inch in front of the bone, and pull it straight backward with as much force as you can without having the tape lift up or slide backward

Posterior Fibular Glide – Part 2

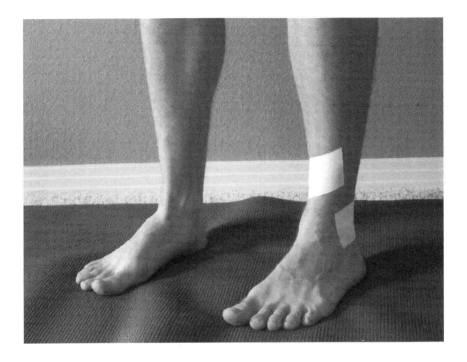

» Keep the tension on the tape, and wrap the tape up your leg. Maintain the tension or pull of the malleolus backward.

» If you feel as though the tape may slip or move, use additional strips of tape over that particular area. If the tape is helpful, you should feel an immediate reduction in pain. Take caution when taping over very swollen ankles.

Ankle Self-Taping Strategies – Kinesiological Taping for Edema (Swelling)

Kinesiological Taping – Step 1

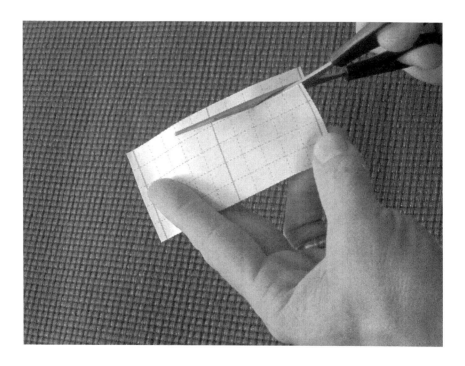

» Turn the Kinesiological tape over and cut along the marked areas approximately quarter inch wide strips. Be sure to leave the last inch or so un-cut.

Kinesiological Taping – Step 2

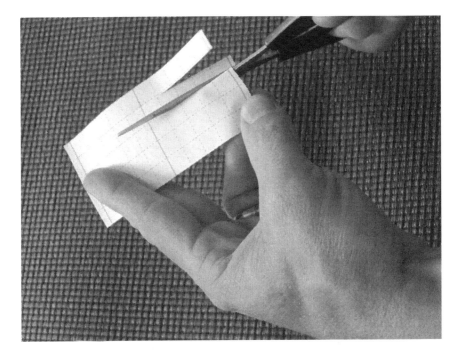

» Be sure to round the corners of the section that remains uncut as that will help insure it that it doesn't catch on your clothing.

Kinesiological Taping - Step 3

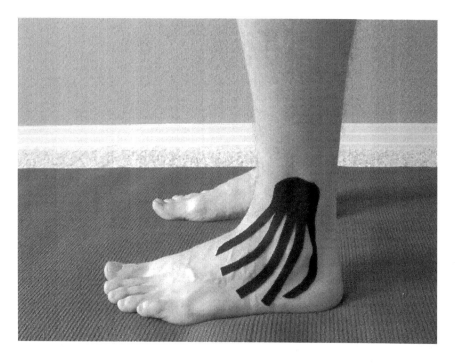

» Apply the anchor (the one inch base) just above the area of most swelling with only slight tension. The strips are to be laid down gently without tension over the area of swelling.

» The Kinesiological tape can be shorter or longer depending on the severity of swelling and what works for you.

Kinesiological Taping – Step 4

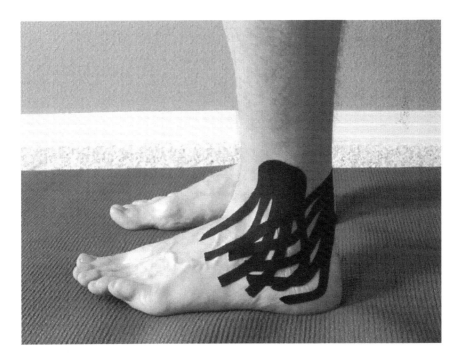

» Depending on the size of the area that is swollen, you can place multiple layers of tape.

» You can even combine other forms of Kinesiological taping (such as the **Circumferential Taping for High Ankle Sprains**) along with this technique.

Ankle Self-Taping Strategies – Circumferential Taping for High Ankle Sprains

Circumferential Taping – Step 1

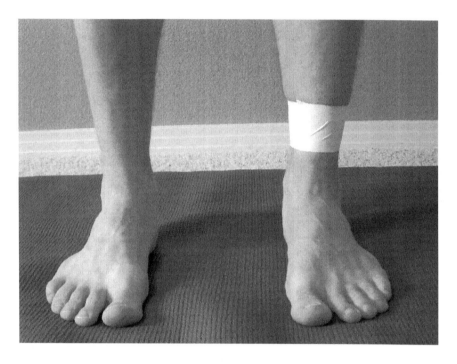

» Sit so that there isn't any weight coming through your foot and ankle. Be sure that your ankle is in a neutral or 90 degree position as if you were standing on it.

» Wrap the ankle with the athletic tape. Only once or twice around the ankle will be necessary. Be sure to wrap just above the ankle malleoli (the bumps on either side of the ankle).

Circumferential Taping – Step 2

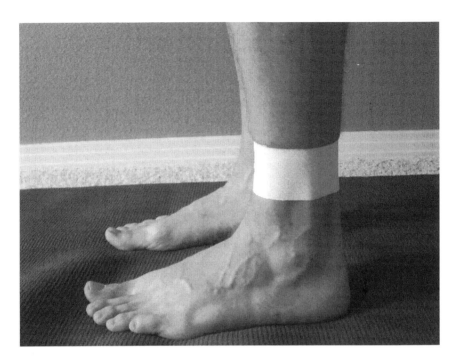

» When wrapping the tape around, there shouldn't be any tension when in a sitting position. The tension will occur once you stand. Be sure that the tape is supportive, but not too tight that you feel numbness or tingling. It shouldn't affect blood flow or cause pain.

» The tape must be worn without fail for at least six weeks for optimal rehabilitation. Don't bear weight on the food without the tape in place.

Skin Care with Taping

WEARING

- **Round the edges prior to application.**

  Rounding the corners helps insure the edges do not catch on clothing and come up prematurely.

- **Prepare the skin initially.**

  Be sure the skin is clean and free from dirt and body oils and lotions. You may want to use a special skin preparation liquid designed to protect the skin. Apply this and allow it to thoroughly dry before applying the tape. Body hair may need to be removed using scissors or clippers, but I do not recommend shaving the area right before application of the tape as this tends to be irritating to the skin.

- **The tape can be worn for several days.**

  Generally the tape can stay on for 4-5 days. Many people are able to wear the tape for a week or so. This may vary with the area being taped and your individual skin. Discuss this with your physical therapist.

- **Shower with the tape on.**

  The tape is water resistant and water proof. You may shower and swim with the tape on. Once out of the water, pat the tape dry.

REMOVAL

- **Remove the tape in the direction of hair growth.**

  If you remove the tape in the opposite direction, it gives a "waxing" type of effect and may pull the hair out.

- **Pull your skin off of the tape.**

  Do not pull the tape off of your skin like a Band-Aid. Peel the tape back on itself and work the skin off of the tape as you peel the tape. Pulling away from the body at a 90 degree angle can pull off layers of skin, which causes redness and irritation.

- **Moisturize the skin.**

  Apply a light moisturizer to the skin as you normally would in your daily care.

Ankle Resistance Exercises – Using the Elastic Exercise Band

As part the sub-acute phase of rehabilitation for ankle sprains and strains, the strength of the muscles that control the ankle and foot must be addressed. The following basic ankle strengthening exercises utilize a **Thera-Band Exercise Band**. The red band is shown and is one of the lighter resistances available. Work on these exercises until you can utilize at least the green band (or beyond for more resistance). The movement may tend to be a bit jittery, but focus on slow controlled motions. The goal is improve your strength and motor control.

- You may have a friend or family member hold the elastic band for you *(and not tie it to a table as shown)*. Please remember if you tie the elastic band, then it must be tied to an object that will not move.

- *With these exercises, remember to move slow and under control.* There should never be more than a mild to moderate increase in discomfort while performing these exercises.

- Start with only the up/down motions (plantarflexion and dorsiflexion). As your pain decreases and your range of motion improves, progress to inversion and eversion with the exercise band. Stop if you experience more than a mild increase in pain levels.

Elastic Band Plantarflexion

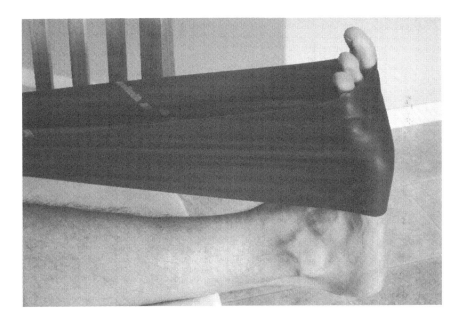

» Start with your foot in a neutral position.

» You may also use the elastic band as a way to stretch your foot up toward you (similar to a standing calf stretch).

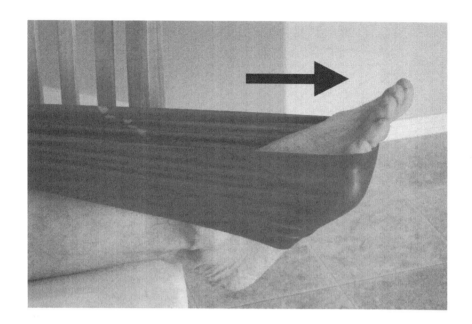

» While seated, use an elastic band attached to your foot and press your foot downward and forward. Return to the starting position slowly and under control.

» Perform 2 sets of 10-15 repetitions, 1-2 times per day on both feet.

» You may have your foot suspended on a chair or stool or with your heel resting on the ground.

Elastic Band Dorsiflexion

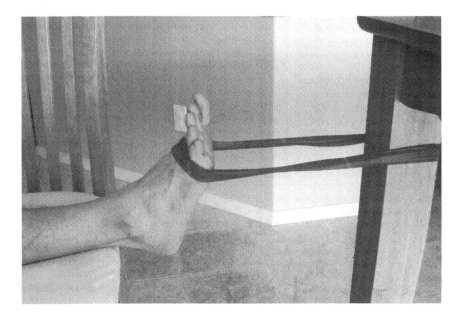

» Start with your foot in a slightly flexed position.

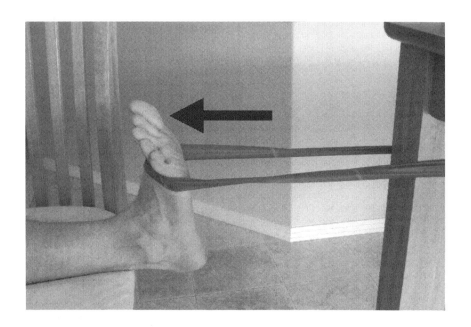

» While seated, use an elastic band attached to your foot and draw your foot upward.

» Perform 2 sets of 10-15 repetitions, 1-2 times per day on both feet.

» You may have your foot suspended on a chair or stool or with your heel resting on the ground.

Elastic Band Inversion

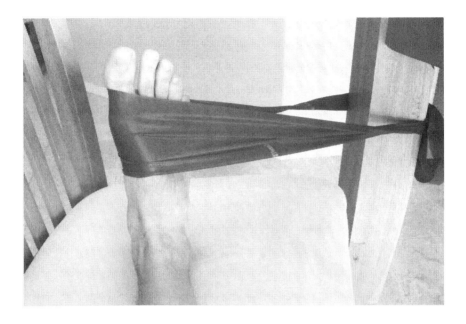

» Start with your foot in a neutral position.

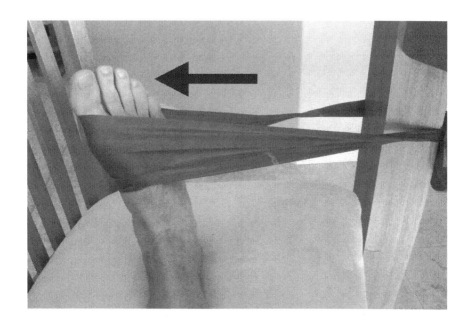

» While seated, use an elastic band attached to your foot and draw your foot inward.

» Perform 2 sets of 10-15 repetitions, 1-2 times per day on both feet.

» You may have your foot suspended on a chair or stool or with your heel resting on the ground.

Elastic Band Eversion

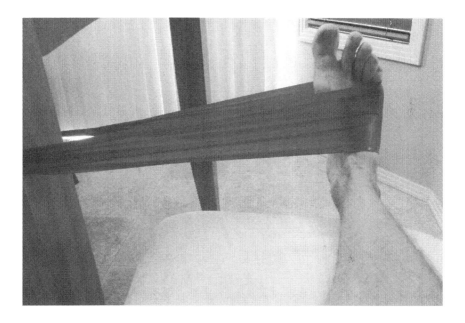

» Start with your foot in a neutral position.

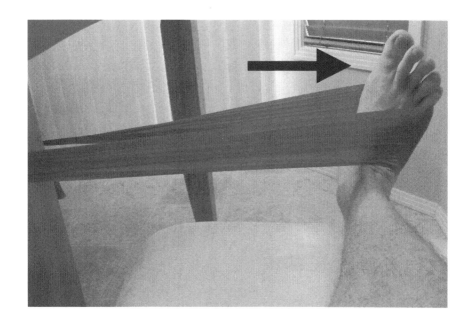

» While seated, use an elastic band attached to your foot and draw your foot outward to the side.

» Perform 2 sets of 10-15 repetitions, 1-2 times per day on both feet.

» You may have your foot suspended on a chair or stool or with your heel resting on the ground.

As your pain improves, you can progress to standing heel and toe raises as long as you don't experience more than a mild increase in pain levels. You may initially start without the step, and then slowly progress by using the step *(as shown below)*. Keep the motions slow and under control. Tape can be worn when performing all exercises.

Heel Raises – Starting Position

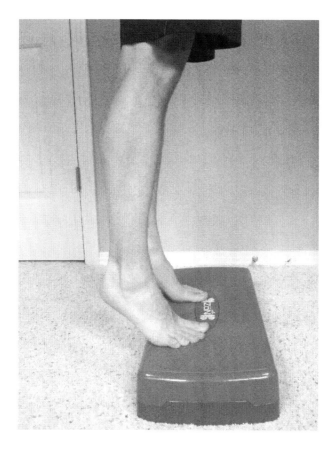

» A key exercise is the heel raise. The emphasis should be on the eccentric control (meaning when the muscle is lengthening or contracting eccentrically).

» In this exercise, the starting position is up on the tip toes. The important component is the slow lowering of the heels. Spend several seconds to lower down the heels. Discontinue this exercise if your pain worsens.

» I recommend **1 second up and taking 5 seconds when coming down.**

Heel Raises – Ending Position

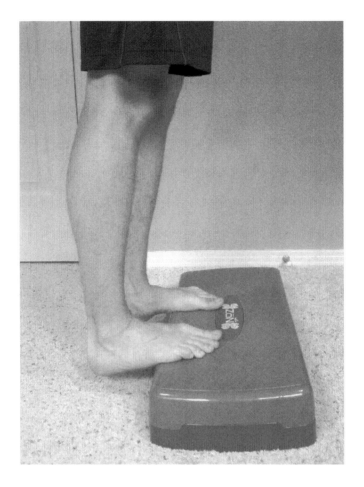

» For normal strength, you should be able to perform 25 repetitions on one foot while using a counter top for minor balance only. As you work on your ankle and plantarflexion strength, start slowly as to not aggravate any painful areas.

» Initially perform with both feet. 10 repetitions at a time, up to 3 sets of 10 repetitions once per day. As your pain level decreases and your strength increases, progress to one foot only and increase the repetitions.

Foot Exercises

It's important to work on the intrinsic muscles of the foot and ankle complex. The following example is one method. You could also work on picking up marbles with your toes.

Foot Intrinsic Muscle Strengthening

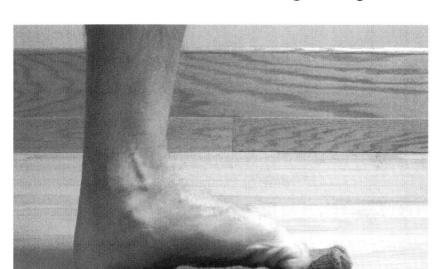

» Place a small towel flat on the floor. A slick non-carpeted floor tends to work best. Try to grab and crinkle the towel by using your toes. Be sure to extend the toes and grab as much as the towel as possible before attempting to grab it again.

» Perform 3 sets of 10 repetitions on each foot once per day

Ankle Resistance Exercises – Other Strengthening

It will be important to increase the weight bearing on the ankle as you work on normal ankle motions during strengthening exercises. Squatting is an excellent method to not only improve general leg strength, but to promote increased ankle mobility. Initially you may not be able to progress down into a full squat. Instead, start with a partial squat while using a chair *(as shown below on the left)*. Start with 2 sets of 10-15 repetitions.

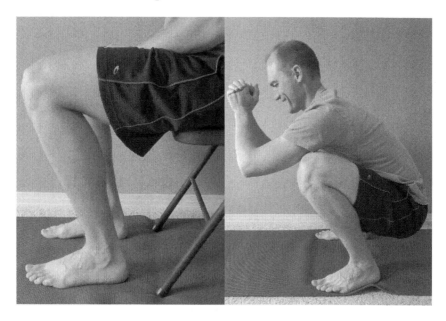

As your range of motion (ROM) improves and your pain reduces, then you can progress your squat deeper *(as shown above on the right)*. Start with 2 sets of 10-15 repetitions. The goal is to promote ROM within a normal movement pattern. (Do not add any weight or resistance during this movement until the **Return to Full Activity and Sport** phase of the rehabilitation.)

Notice the difference between the ankle's ROM during a partial versus a full squat. Most importantly, keep your knee in alignment with your second toe in order to insure proper positioning for your knee and ankle.

You may also find that utilizing the posterior fibular glide taping technique is helpful in order to improve your ankle's range of motion as well as your ability to walk normally and to squat. (Please refer to **Ankle Self-Taping Strategies – Posterior Fibular Glide**.) *Apply the tape prior to performing weight bearing exercises including: walking; toe raises; and squatting.*

If you are recovering from a high ankle sprain and you are utilizing the circumferential taping, be sure it's intact for all weight bearing activities and exercises. (Please refer to **Ankle Self-Taping Strategies – Circumferential Taping for High Ankle Sprains**.)

Initial Balance and Proprioception Exercises

Balance and proprioception exercises are an important component to the rehabilitation program. Not only will working on balance help you to progress through the rehabilitation and recovery, but more importantly, it can help you to reduce the risk of re-injury.

As the pain subsides and your balance improves, you may need to increase the difficulty level when standing on one foot. As you progress, balance will become of greater importance (this is addressed in more detail during the final stage of recovery).

Standing on One Foot with Finger Tips

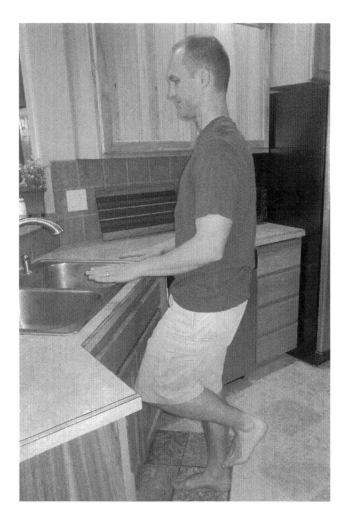

» Initially, you may need to use your hand (or a finger) on a counter top for added support.

» Don't allow yourself to wobble or wiggle too much.

» Use your fingertips as needed to maintain balance. You shouldn't experience more than a mild increase in pain or discomfort during this exercise.

Standing on One Foot

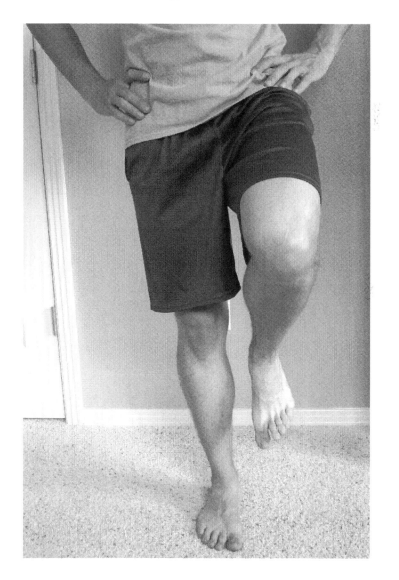

» The ability to hold for 30 seconds with eyes open during the first time, and then closed during the second time, is considered normal.

» Perform for 30 seconds, 2-3 repetitions per day.

Other Treatment Options

There are many options for additional treatment methods and modalities in the sub-acute phase. Each treatment modality has its place and use depending on your rehabilitation process. Recovery can vary from one person to another. During this phase, you may choose to seek additional rehabilitation assistance.

The purpose of this book is to help guide you through a self-treatment plan that allows for a safe return to activity. In most ankle sprain cases, one can effectively work through a rehabilitation protocol. However, it may be warranted or desired to ask for additional assistance. Rehabilitation professionals have different strengths and biases on how to assist with rehabilitation, so there are many treatment options available.

Other treatment options include:

- **LOCAL MODALITIES.** Local modalities are used to assist with pain reduction and the natural healing response via an increase in energy modulation or nutrient delivery. This includes: electrical stimulation; ultrasound; infra-red light; use of magnets or magnetic fields; and temperature modulation (such as contrast baths). These modalities have short-term benefits that can assist with the earlier introduction of other longer lasting techniques (such as an exercise prescription that includes strength, balance, and range of motion exercises).

  While many clients will feel the immediate benefits from this form of passive treatment, it's best to think of these modalities similarly to analgesic and/or NSAID medications.

It's a method of pain relief or inflammation reduction that provides short-term relief which allows you to continue living as comfortably as possible until you have recovered.

- **MANUAL TECHNIQUES.** Hands-on manual techniques can be beneficial initially to help reduce pain levels as well as edema and swelling while promoting normal range of motion. Some techniques may even promote improved nutrient delivery and exchange to aid in the healing response. Examples of manual techniques include: soft tissue mobilization; massage; IASTM (instrument assisted soft tissue mobilization); joint mobilization techniques; acupuncture; and dry needling techniques.

In the case of ankle sprains/strains, joint stiffness or laxity can be a complication associated with injury to the joint and adjacent muscle, tendon, and ligament. It can be beneficial to have a physical therapist that is highly skilled in regaining full joint motion via a range of skillful hands-on techniques to assist in your recovery, but it's not necessary in every case. If you consult with a physical therapist or rehabilitation professional, the ultimate goal is to provide the **safest, quickest, and most-effective solution** to address any particular issue when guiding you through the rehabilitation process.

The **American Physical Therapy Association** offers a wonderful resource to help find a physical therapist in your area. In most states, you can seek physical therapy advice without a medical doctor's referral (although it may be a good idea to seek your physician's opinion as well).

- **EXERCISE PRESCRIPTION.** Research has shown that exercise prescription is the most effective method to hasten recovery, reduce pain, and improve your post-injury function. Exercises may include: specific stretching exercises; strengthening exercises; localized (directed at the site of injury) and global (for example, core stability and adjacent muscle groups); barbell training; proprioceptive and balance retraining; biomechanics correction; and functional or sport-specific rehabilitation.

Rehabilitation Recap for the Sub-Acute Ankle Sprain

Continue with **PRICE** (**P**rotect, **R**est, **I**ce, **C**ompression, and **E**levation) on an as needed basis.

As you progress into full range of motion (ROM) in the ankle, **rest** and take **pain relieving measures** as needed. Focus on getting full dorsiflexion ROM first. Don't forget that your body needs **healthy food and nutrients** to help it heal. Consider **supplementation** to help insure that your body has the necessary nutrients for a speedy recovery.

Toward the end of the intermediate phase, you should be walking normally without an assistive device. There will likely be some swelling after a long day or heavy use. Pain should be minimal. You may continue to wear compression stockings during this time. Continue with taping techniques in general. *If you're utilizing the circumferential taping technique, continue with it for at least six to eight weeks regardless of symptoms.*

It's time to progress into the final stage of rehabilitation once you have returned to near normal walking. Your pain levels should be relatively low. You should be able to complete the basic exercises (as demonstrated throughout this section, **Intermediate (Sub-Acute) Phase of Rehabilitation**) without significant pain or difficulty. The final stage of rehabilitation includes a full return to daily activities and eventually, all sport or athletic activities.

During the sub-acute phase, you should be as active as you can be, but don't over stress the injury. You should be able to return to all normal activities of daily living. You may still be intermittently wearing a brace during more active times or times of being on your feet without a break.

Prior to progressing out of the sub-acute phase of rehabilitation and into a return to full activity and sport, insure the following:

- You should be able to stand on the injured side on one leg without pain.

- There is only intermittent swelling in and around the ankle and lower leg. It typically occurs at the end of the day or after prolonged activity.

- You are able to lightly jog without an increase of pain or a feeling of significant ankle instability.

- You don't have any other injury that would require medical management.

Depending on severity and actual tissues injured, the sub-acute phase of rehabilitation for an ankle sprain can last one or two weeks up to six weeks on average. If you are unsure on how to progress your rehabilitation, be sure to ask for help.

RETURN TO FULL ACTIVITY AND SPORT

As a physical therapist, I find that the most exciting part of a person's rehabilitation is the full return to function, activity or sport. Countless variations of exercises and activities are performed while working toward restoring the full functional use of the ankle.

Each individual will progress through a rehabilitation plan differently. Therefore, no treatment plan will be exactly alike, but similar. For discussion purposes, I address a generic treatment plan which should be modified for your personal needs, activity level or specific sport needs.

In this final stage of rehabilitation, you will progress to normal daily activities, including any athletic endeavors. This is also when you work toward limiting any future re-occurrence of the sprain.

At this stage in recovery, you should be able to:

- Walk normally and pain-free.
- Lightly jog without significant pain or a feeling of instability.

Running and more active side-to-side movements may still cause pain. Although not contra-indicated, these types of activities should be limited (unless you're wearing a lace-up or slip-on style brace or utilizing taping techniques to help with stability).

The initial portion of this stage of rehabilitation is focused on improving ankle and foot strength and stability as well as addressing any balance deficits. This process begins with static based exercises and activities. Ultimately, it progresses into dynamic strength, balance, and mobility activities. How rapidly one progresses in this phase is highly variable. **The key is to progress at your own pace.**

If you begin to experience increasing pain, feelings of ankle instability, and/or sensations that your ankle may "roll" or sprain again, then you need to taper down your activity level and continue with the strategies outlined in the **Intermediate (Sub-Acute) Phase of Rehabilitation**. After the pain subsides, continue to focus on the activities that didn't cause pain or discomfort previously.

The following treatment plan includes exercises for strength and balance as well as mobility drills and full athletic simulation drills. Each category is listed in an easiest to most challenging format. You shouldn't progress to the next exercise until the first one is mastered (performed pain-free with proper technique and motor control).

Strength

- Continue with the **Ankle Resistance Exercises – Using the Elastic Exercise Band,** but progress to a more resistant **Thera-Band Exercise Band.** The red band is one of the lighter resistances available. Work on these exercises until you can utilize at least the green band (or beyond for more resistance).

- **Heel/Toe Raises** – For normal strength, you should be able to perform 25 heel raises in a row with only minimal fingertip assistance on a counter top. A normal amount of calf strength would be considered once you can perform 25 heel raises using one foot only *(as demonstrated on the following page)*.

Heel Raises

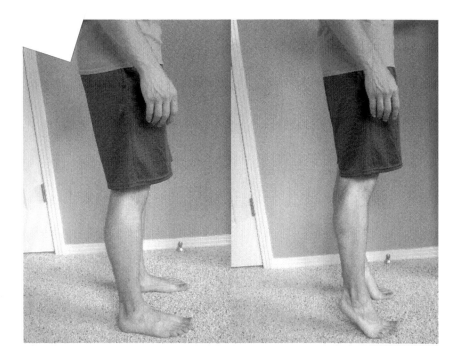

» Initially start with your feet flat on the ground. As this becomes easy, progress to using a step.

» 10 repetitions at a time, up to 3 sets of 10 repetitions once per day.

Heel Raises – Starting Position

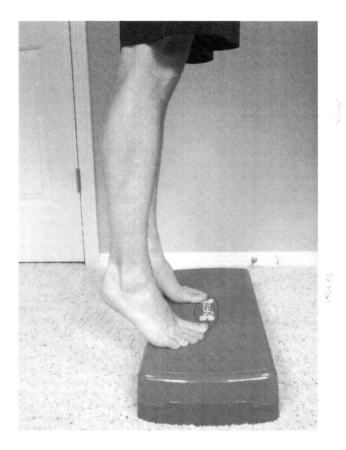

» A key exercise is the heel raise. The emphasis should be on the eccentric control (meaning when the muscle is lengthening or contracting eccentrically).

» In this exercise, the starting position is up on the tip toes. The important component is the slow lowering of the heels. Spend several seconds to lower down the heels. Discontinue this exercise if your pain worsens.

» I recommend **1 second up and taking 5 seconds when coming down.**

Heel Raises - Ending Position

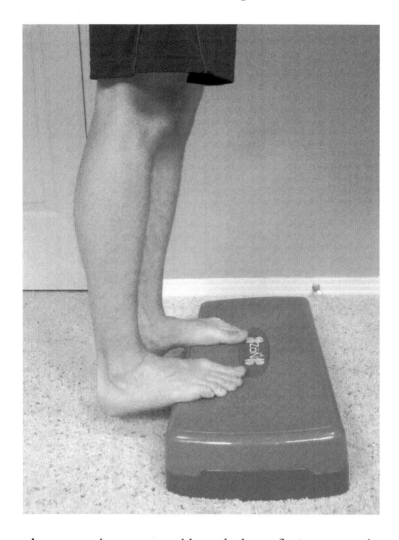

» As you work on your ankle and plantarflexion strength, start slowly as to not aggravate the painful area.

» Initially perform with both feet. 10 repetitions at a time, up to 3 sets of 10 repetitions once per day. As your pain level decreases and your strength increases, progress to one foot only and increase the repetitions.

Heel Raises - One Leg

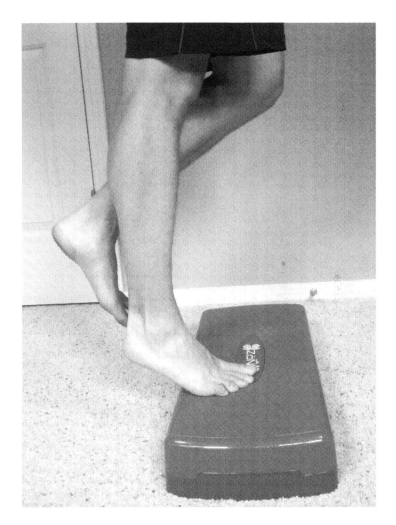

» For normal strength, you should be able to perform 25 repetitions on one foot while using a counter top for minor balance only. As you work on your ankle and plantarflexion strength, start slowly as to not aggravate the painful area.

» 10 repetitions at a time, up to 3 sets of 10 repetitions once per day.

One Leg Partial Squat

This particular exercise will work on the strength of the calf and ankle as well as the quadriceps and hip.

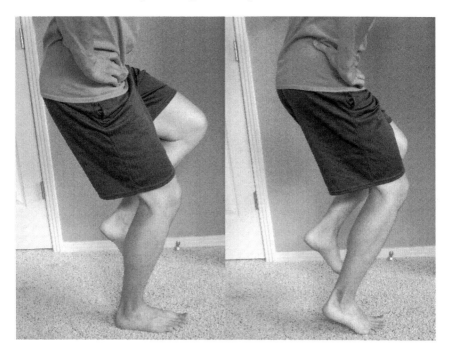

» Initially you may need to use your finger tips on a counter or a wall.

» To increase the difficulty, do not use your hands for balance. The one leg squat on your tip toes is a harder variation which involves more calf muscle activation.

» Start with 2 sets of 10 repetitions, then progress to 3 sets of 10 repetitions.

Clock/Star Exercise

» When performed properly, this exercise works on strength as well as balance and proprioception. Stand on your affected (injured) foot and attempt to touch your tip toe of the non-affected side as far out as you can reach. Bring your foot back to the center or starting point according to the hands on a clock. For example, 1 o'clock to 6 o'clock (clock-wise) or 12 'o clock to 6 o' clock (counter clock-wise) depending on which foot is affected. Perform the routine between three to five times **slowly**.

Single Leg Balance with Mini Squat
(The Star Drill)

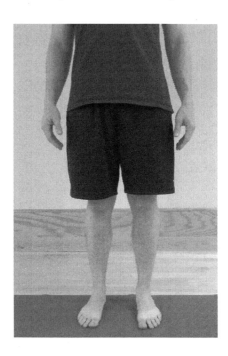

» To address all aspects of how the knee functions, we must also address balance and stability. You will start this exercise on two legs, and then by standing on your injured leg. You will slowly move the non-injured leg as described below. Try to maintain your balance and reach your non-injured leg as far out as you can. You will eventually bend your injured knee as you reach further. The goal is maintain balance, reach as far as you can, and keep your patella (knee cap) straight ahead by tracking in line with your second toe.

» You will perform the exercises below in succession. Touch your toe, and then return to standing on one foot. Repeat with the next position. You will proceed through all three positions for 5-10 times before repeating with your other leg.

The Star Drill
Reaching Forward

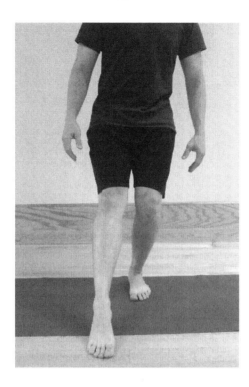

» Standing on your injured leg, slowly move the non-injured leg forward. The goal is to maintain your balance, reach your non-injured leg as far out as you can, and keep your patella (knee cap) straight ahead by tracking in line with your second toe. You will eventually bend your injured knee as you reach further.

» You will touch only one time, and then return the leg to the starting position (but stay standing on one leg only). Proceed to the next position. Just barely touch a tip toe.

» Proceed through all three positions for 5-10 times before repeating with your other leg.

The Star Drill
Reaching Sideways

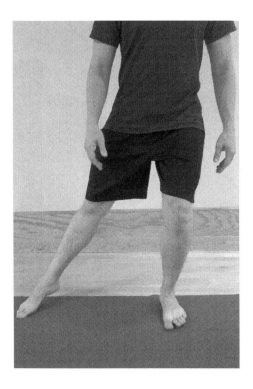

» Standing on your injured leg, slowly move the non-injured leg sideways. The goal is to maintain your balance, reach your non-injured leg as far out as you can, and keep your patella (knee cap) straight ahead by tracking in line with your second toe. You will eventually bend your injured knee as you reach further. Just barely touch a tip toe.

» You will touch only one time, and then return the leg to the starting position (but stay standing on one leg only). Proceed to the next position.

» Proceed through all three positions for 5-10 times before repeating with your other leg.

The Star Drill
Reaching Backwards

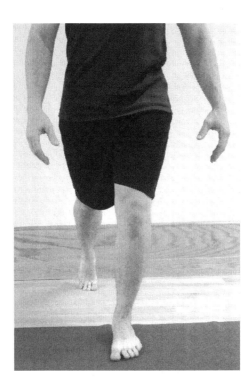

» Standing on your injured leg, slowly move the non-injured leg backward. The goal is to maintain your balance, reach your non-injured leg as far out as you can, and keep your patella (knee cap) straight ahead by tracking in line with your second toe. You will eventually bend your injured knee as you reach further. Just barely touch a tip toe.

» You will touch only one time, and then return the leg to the starting position (but stay standing on one leg only). Proceed to the next position.

» Proceed through all three positions for 5-10 times before repeating with your other leg.

One Legged Twist – Starting Position

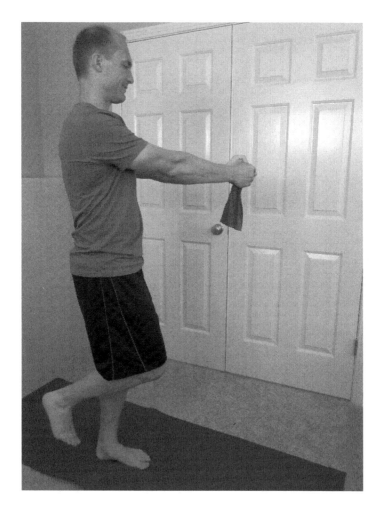

» Attach an exercise band to a door or post. Stand on your injured leg, so that when you rotate, it will be away from the doorway. As shown, I'm standing on my left foot with my left shoulder sideway to the door. I rotate toward my right side.

» The goal is to maintain a good upright posture and to maintain your balance on the affected leg as you slowly rotate your body against resistance.

One Legged Twist

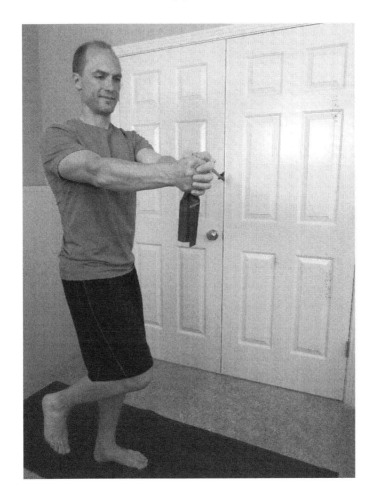

» Perform this exercise slowly at first and maintain your balance and control. Initially, you may not get a full twisting motion. As you improve, attempt to increase the range of motion of the twist.

» As you progress, also perform this exercise quickly, but always in control of the motion.

» Perform 3 sets of 10 repetitions, and 3-5 times per week.

Weight Training

Once the pain has subsided, swelling and stability has improved, and you are working toward a full return to sport, you should also return to your full weight lifting routine. As with returning to lifting after any injury, start slowly and see how each lift affects you and feels.

The most obvious lifts to return to first include squats and deadlifts. Although these lifts typically have you lifting the most weight, they are performed on a steady surface without much foot movement. The downside to the squat is that it requires ankle mobility. You may need to limit the depth of the squat until you can reach full range of motion (ROM) without pain.

As with any training session, warm up prior to adding load to the work sets. Working with the bar and/or the bar with a light load (such as 25% of your one rep max), move through the full ROM of the lift. Assess how your ankle feels. As it improves, slowly taper up the amount of weight lifted.

Once you are performing full ROM when squatting and your ankle is tolerating quick movements, start with more technical lifts that require the feet to move. These include the clean, snatch, push press, and the split jerk. Again, start with a light load to insure that your ankle is ready to progress into the heavier lifts.

By the time you return to full sport and activity, you should also be returning to full training. This is likely going to be a process that evolves over a few weeks as you continue to work through other aspects of your rehabilitation. As with all injuries, the recovery process will look slightly different for everyone.

Balance and Proprioception Drills

There are many options to work on balance and proprioception. Always start with the easier versions and progress to the more difficult options. Get creative! Here are some of my favorites.

- **STAND ON ONE FOOT** – A 30 second hold with eyes open during the first time, then closed during the second time, is considered normal.

- **STAND ON ONE FOOT ON A PILLOW** – Begin with a 30 second hold for two to three repetitions. *To progress this further, stand on a foam pad (or a Wobble Board or Bosu Balance Trainer that most health clubs have).* As you progress, stand on the pillow and perform the **Clock/Star Exercise** *(as demonstrated in Strength)*.

- **STAND ON ONE FOOT ON A WATER NOODLE** – This exercise challenges your balance due to the softer surface and the narrow water noodle. It also challenges the side-to-side stability of the ankle, which is the weakest area, yet the most critical, with a lateral ankle sprain. Perform a 30 second hold for two to three repetitions.

- Other activities to increase balance and proprioceptive response in the ankle and lower leg include:
  - Stand on one foot and bounce a ball against a wall.
  - Stand on a Wobble Board, Bosu Balance Trainer, or other unstable surface.

Balancing on One Foot

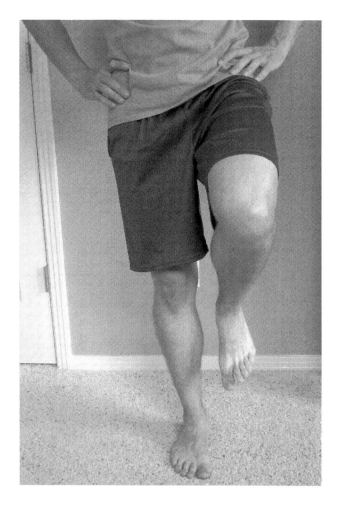

» While standing near a counter top, stand on one foot. Use your hands on the counter top only as needed to maintain your balance. Maintain a proper upright posture. The softer the surface you stand on, the more difficult the balance will be.

» Hold for 30 seconds, and 3 repetitions per side. *(If your balance is very poor initially, please stand near a counter or sink for safety.)*

Balancing on One Foot – Soft Surface

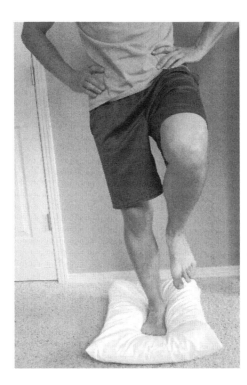

» Proper balance is a critical component when rehabilitating an ankle sprain. Work on standing on one foot. Once you have mastered it, increase the difficulty level by adding a pillow or standing on any type of softer surface, such as grass, a foam pad, air disc or Bosu Balance Trainer.

» For normal balance, you should be able to stand on one foot for 30 seconds with both eyes open and with both eyes closed on the firm ground. *(If your balance is very poor initially, please stand near a counter or sink for safety.)*

Balancing on One Foot – Lateral Instability

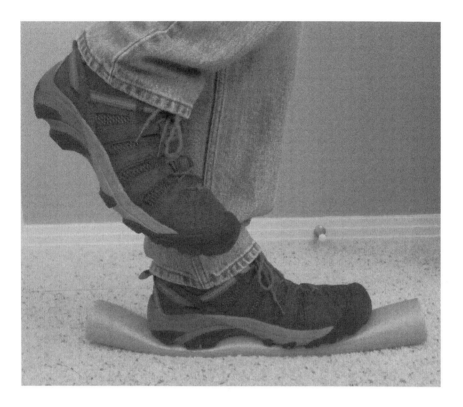

» Regaining normal lateral/side to side balance is a critical component when rehabilitating an ankle sprain. After you have mastered standing on one foot, progress to standing on a water noodle. Initially start with shoes on, and then progress to bare feet.

» Hold for 30 seconds, and 3 repetitions per side.

» *(If your balance is very poor initially, please stand near a counter or sink for safety.)*

Clock/Star Exercise – Lateral Instability

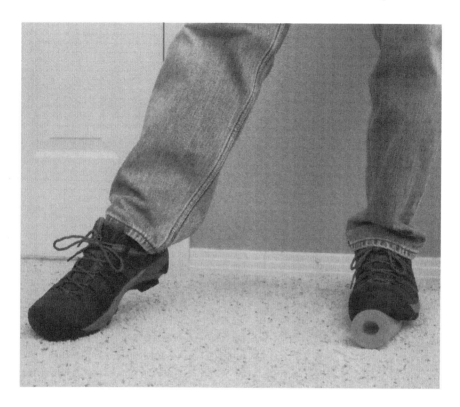

» After you can easily perform the **Clock/Star Exercise** and you can easily balance on the water noodle *in shoes and bare feet*, combine the two exercises by performing the **Clock/Star Exercise** while balancing on the water noodle.

» Proceed through all three positions for 5-10 times before repeating with your other leg. Perform in shoes and bare feet.

» *(If your balance is very poor initially, please stand near a counter or sink for safety.)*

Returning to Mobility Drills

During this phase, you are well on your way to mastering the static balance exercises. You may initially continue to wear your lace-up or slip-on style brace (if you have been wearing one). Depending on how long it has been since the initial injury, you may continue to wear your circumferential tape. (Six weeks is optimal for rehabilitation.) Ultimately, you should be to perform these exercises without additional support. If you are uncertain, start with the brace or tape on, and then progress out of it as you gain confidence.

Initially, start with **forward and backward movements** and progress from a **walk to a jog to a sprint**.

Mobility Drills include:

- **JUMP ROPING**
- **SIDE STEPPING** – Progress the speed as pain allows and only if you're *not* experiencing a feeling of instability.
- **KARAOKE OR GRAPEVINE** – Walk or run sideways while alternating the placement of the foot either in front or behind the other.
- **HOPPING** – Side to side and front to back on one leg.
- **SPRINT LADDER** – A number of agility drills can be performed with the sprint ladder. Search YouTube and pick your favorite video which closely mimics the footwork desired for your particular sport or activity.

- **SHORT SIDE-TO-SIDE WIND SPRINTS** – When sprinting, touch your hand to the ground at each change of direction.

Full Athletic Simulation Drills and Return to Sport

Depending on your sport of choice, it's time to return to your sport specific training drills. Initially, start at 50-75% of your normal speed. As you gain confidence with how your ankle is feeling and moving, taper up the speed until you are able to perform the activity at full speed.

During this initial return to athletic simulation drills, you may still require additional support. You may wear a lace-up brace or have a professional tape your ankle for support. Additional support should only be used temporarily and with the intention of progressing from using it as your ankle can tolerate.

Once you are able to perform all athletic simulation drills at full speed and you have full confidence in your ankle, it's time to return to full sporting activities. During this final return to sport phase, it's important to remember that your ankle will likely require an additional warm up to insure it is ready to perform at a high level. Perform the basic range of motion drills followed by toe raises and partial squats in addition to some balance drills. Be sure to warm up so that the nervous system is "awake", but don't over fatigue the area.

Rehabilitation Recap for the Return to Full Activity and Sport

First, insure that you have met the requirements for progressing out of the sub-acute phase of rehabilitation and into a return to full activity and sport. You should be able to perform all sport related drills correctly without pain or instability before returning to actual competitive play.

Don't forget that your body needs **healthy food and nutrients** to help it heal. Continue with any **supplementation** in order to insure that your body has the necessary nutrients for at least several weeks as you return to full activity and sporting endeavors.

Prior to progressing out of this phase of rehabilitation into a full return to sport and all activities, insure the following:

- You have normal balance for your daily and sports needs without pain.

- You can perform all of your specific sport agility drills at full speed without pain or instability.

- Your ankle feels at least back to its prior "normal" status, if not better than it did prior to injury.

- When hopping laterally (sideways) on the injured leg, can you in three hops travel as far toward the injured side as you can hopping on your good leg toward the other side (good side)?

The return to sport and activity phase of an ankle sprain can last multiple weeks. It depends on your activity level and which tasks that you need your ankle to perform. Depending on the severity of the injury and actual tissues injured, you may be several weeks post injury or twelve or more weeks post injury.

The key to full recovery is to insure that your ankle is performing all desired tasks under a controlled environment prior to progressing to an unknown environment (like during the field of play/sport). Don't skip the different phases of recovery or the different aspects of the rehabilitation: range of motion (ROM), strength, and balance. Each component is critical to proper ankle functioning and will be required as you progress back into full activity. Always "test" the ankle in simulation drills prior to returning to full athletics and activity. Continue with your ankle rehabilitation protocol for at least two weeks after your return to full activity in order to help prevent future injury and reoccurrences.

PREVENTION

Whether you have a history of ankle sprains or just want to prevent one, the treatments outlined can be adapted as a preventative approach. Although I participate in very ankle demanding activities (including trail running, hiking, and obstacle course racing), I haven't suffered an ankle injury in over twenty years. I attribute this to implementing a prevention strategy.

Ankle sprains can reoccur frequently if you don't take the necessary time to rehabilitate the injury. If you are recovering from an injury, don't skip the rehabilitation protocol. Even if you have returned to most activities, keep working through the rehabilitation plan.

The key components to preventing ankle sprains and strains are **strength** and **balance**. Strength is a broad term. In the case of a lower extremity injury as well as an ankle injury, the key is maintaining adequate strength in the foot ankle complex all the way up the chain from the knee to the hip to the core. The core and lower extremity chain work together for all mobility. If there is a weak spot in the chain, whether it is in the hip or the ankle, your risk of injury will increase.

Balance is a general term indicating the integration of the neuro-musculoskeletal system which includes one's eyesight, vestibular system, proprioception, muscle strength, and neurological system. With proper training, all of these body systems will function at a high level and help you avoid injury.

Strength

Your body must always have sufficient strength to perform your desired task or sport as well as maintain adequate reserves. This means that you always need at least enough strength to do whatever it is that you are asking your body to perform. Ideally, you're strong enough in order to insure that if something goes wrong, then your body has the strength to handle it. Often an injury will occur when the task is harder or takes more effort or strength than the body can produce.

Barbell training is the most effective method to increase strength due the progressive load on the skeletal system and the muscle pull which is exerted on the bone. It increases your body's margin for error when illness or injury occurs. With proper guidance and the right exercise prescription/dosage, nearly everyone can improve in strength and benefit from weight training. I recommend that you read ***Starting Strength: Basic Barbell Training*** by Mark Rippetoe.

Resistance training (other than through barbell training) can also be beneficial. An example of resistance training would be any type of pushing or pulling exercise that exerts a force on the muscle, which causes it to work harder than it would normally. The key to all training is that the system must be properly overloaded to produce the desired effect. Too little, and you will not receive a positive benefit. Too much, and you risk injury. This overload principle must guide all exercise routines if there is to be actual success and benefit from the program. Although any properly dosed/prescribed form of resistive exercise would be beneficial, the most effective exercises either activate large muscle groups and/or load the skeletal system. Examples include squats, lunges, and dead lifts.

In order to prevent ankle sprains/strains in general, work on your strength. Being stronger will always better prepare you for the terrain you will run on and the obstacles and/or sports performed. Weight training will also help to increase your body's margin for error when illness or injury occurs. To quote Mark Rippetoe, "Stronger people are harder to kill than weak people and more useful in general."

As part of preparing your body to generate a rapid force, I also highly recommend plyometric style training which should be sport or activity specific. If your sport requires jumping, then plyometric jumping off of a box should be part of your training routine. If your sport requires side-to-side movements, then sideways bounding should be part of your routine. Always keep in mind the activity that you are training for and add the appropriate sport specific training.

Balance

When addressing balance for prevention or sports performance, it's important that you look at all areas of the sport or activity you will be participating in and add balance drills that require a higher difficulty level than what is typically found during the event. If your event requires one legged activities, then time should be spent on one legged balance activities.

Manipulate the different variables and components of balance. For example, when you're standing on one foot, move your head up and down and left and right. While standing on one foot, jump up and down or throw a ball back and forth. Try standing on one foot while standing on a water noodle and throwing a ball. Please refer to **Balance and Proprioception Drills** for suggestions on how to improve your balance (particularly in regard to proprioceptive balance).

During balance training, you're attempting to work on different aspects of balance such as proprioception or vestibular function. This is not the time to develop strength. People often confuse the two and attempt to work on "functional" strength by trying to do something fancy like squat on a Bosu Balance Trainer.

If your intention is to become stronger, then work on strength training, which should include barbell training. For example, squat with your feet on a solid surface so that you can generate maximum force (not on a Bosu Balance Trainer). If your intention is on balance training, then by all means use the Bosu Balance Trainer. Just keep the two types of training separate.

The best way to improve balance is to embrace your inner child. Balance on curbs, jump up and down on stumps, and vary the terrain. Even close your eyes and spin or jump up and down. By making play a part of your life and routine, you stimulate all aspects of your balance and engage all your systems (eyesight, vestibular, proprioception, neurological, and muscular).

When running or hiking on uneven terrain, be sure that you're utilizing the natural ability of the foot to bend, maneuver, and contort over uneven terrain. If you land with a mid-foot strike, your foot has a much greater ability to adapt to its terrain versus landing heel or toe first.

Training and practice of these balance activities will help you to avoid ankle sprains. If you have already experienced a sprain, then you're more likely to experience one again. However, you can significantly reduce your risk of another ankle sprain by implementing these exercises and strategies.

CONCLUSION

The purpose of this book is to help guide you through a self-treatment plan that allows for a safe return to activity. Your progression through rehabilitation will vary as its dependent on the severity of your injury. Each person and injury is different.

The key to full recovery is to insure that your ankle is performing all desired tasks under a controlled environment prior to progressing to an unknown environment (like during the field of play/sport). Don't skip the different phases of recovery or the different aspects of the rehabilitation: range of motion (ROM), strength, and balance. Each component is critical to proper ankle functioning and will be required as you progress back into full activity. Always "test" the ankle in simulation drills prior to returning to full athletics and activity.

Continue with your ankle rehabilitation protocol for at least two weeks after your return to full activity in order to help prevent future injury and reoccurrences. Then progress into a long term prevention strategy.

In most ankle sprain cases, one can effectively work through a rehabilitation protocol. However, it may be warranted or desired to ask for additional assistance.

Contact a sports medicine physical therapist or athletic trainer if:

- You continue to experience pain and swelling.

- You are struggling with progressing through any of the different phases of rehabilitation.

- You require an accelerated time table for recovery (or return to competition).

There are many different treatment modalities (electrical stimulation, manual techniques, and other taping methods) which can assist in recovery when properly utilized. (Please refer to **Other Treatment Options**.)

The **American Physical Therapy Association** offers a wonderful resource to help find a physical therapist in your area. In most states, you can seek physical therapy advice without a medical doctor's referral (although it may be a good idea to seek your physician's opinion as well).

RESOURCE GUIDE

⊤ʜᴇPHYSICAL THERAPYADVISOR
Empowering You to Reach Your Optimal Health!

NOTE: Throughout this guide, I reference books, products, supplements, topical agents, and web sites that I personally use and recommend to my family, friends, clients, and patients (for use in the clinical setting). For your reference and convenience, these resources are listed at: **www.thephysicaltherapyadvisor.com/resource-guide**

Some of the links are "affiliate links." This means if you click on the link and purchase the item, I will receive an affiliate commission **at no extra cost to you**. I recommend them because they are helpful and useful, not because of the small commission I make if you decide to buy something.

BOOKS

- *Starting Strength: Basic Barbell Training* by Mark Rippetoe

PRODUCTS

- EDGE Mobility Bands

- KT TAPE
- Mummy Tape
- RockTape Kinesiology Tape
- Rogue Fitness VooDoo X Bands
- Thera-Band Exercise Band

SUPPLEMENTS

- Mag Glycinate
- Mt. Capra CapraColostrum
- Mt. Capra CapraFlex
- Thorne Research Magnesium Citrate
- Tissue Rejuvenator by Hammer Nutrition

TOPICAL AGENTS

- Ancient Minerals Magnesium Bath Flakes
- Arnica Rub
- Biofreeze
- Epsoak Epson Salt

WEB SITES

- American Physical Therapy Association
- The Physical Therapy Advisor

MORE SELF-TREATMENT EBOOKS

My goal as a physical therapist and author is to help proactive adults of all ages to understand how to safely self-treat and manage common musculoskeletal, neurological, and mobility related conditions in a timely manner so they can reach their optimal health. With the cost of healthcare on the rise and no sign of that trend improving, it will become even more necessary to have quality self-treatment education available.

Other eBooks you may be interested in:

Treating Low Back Pain (LBP) during Exercise and Athletics

In this eBook, I share very specific strategies for general LBP prevention among athletes such as sport enthusiasts, CrossFitters, weightlifters, and runners. These principles are helpful for anyone participating in athletics as well as those implementing a healthy lifestyle. You'll learn how to address specific causes of LBP as well as the best practices on how to prevent and self-treat when you experience an episode of LBP. In this step-by-step LBP rehabilitation guide (complete with photos and detailed exercise descriptions), you will discover how to implement prevention and rehabilitation strategies.

Preventing and Treating Overtraining Syndrome

In this eBook, I show you how to recognize the risk factors and symptoms of Overtraining Syndrome (OTS). You'll learn how to utilize prevention strategies to help you develop a personal training strategy that will allow you to push past your limits and prior plateau points in order to reach a state of what is known as overreaching (your body's ability to "supercompensate"). This will speed up your results, so that you can train harder and more effectively than ever before! In addition, learn how to use the foam roller (complete with photos and detailed exercise descriptions) as part of a health optimization program, recovery program, rest day or treatment modality.

Be sure to stay tuned for upcoming eBooks including my guide to **Running an Injury-Free Marathon**.

STAY CONNECTED!

THE**PHYSICAL THERAPY**ADVISOR
Empowering You to Reach Your Optimal Health!

When you subscribe to my e-mail newsletter, I will send you blog posts on how to maximize your health, self-treat those annoying orthopaedic injuries, and gracefully age. To thank you for subscribing, you will automatically gain access to all of my FREE resources, including a FREE CHAPTER from my eBook, **Treating Low Back Pain during Exercise and Athletics**.

Be sure to join our growing community on Facebook by liking **The Physical Therapy Advisor** where you will receive additional health and lifestyle information!

Please submit your feedback, comments, and/or questions to:

contact@thePhysicalTherapyAdvisor.com

Made in the USA
Monee, IL
11 August 2020

37972588R00068